Pharmacy Dilution Calculations

By Babir Malik

About the author

Babir studied pharmacy at the University of Bradford and graduated in 2007 (after previously studying Biomedical Sciences at the same university). He joined Weldricks Pharmacy as a summer student in 2005, undertook his pre-reg with them and has stayed with them ever since.

Babir is now the Weldricks Pre-reg and Pharmacy Student Lead and Weldricks Teacher Practitioner, at the University of Bradford. He is also the Green Light Campus Northern Pre-Reg Lead, PCPA National Pre-reg Lead, Charity Ambassador for Pharmacist Support, Associate Fellow at HEA, as well as a tutor on the Royal Pharmaceutical Society Pre-Registration Conferences.

Babir currently practices as a relief pharmacist for Weldricks. In June 2016, the pharmacy that he co-managed at the time was awarded the Chemist and Druggist Medicines Optimisation Award for their innovative Local Pharmaceutical Service Intervention Service. He is a Chemist and Druggist Clinical Advisory Board Member.

As a Teacher Practitioner, his role includes being the MPharm Calculations Lead. Furthermore, Babir undertook a 10-week secondment as a Clinical Commissioning Group Pharmacist in North Lincolnshire early in 2016. He is also an OnTrack question writer and reviewer and is on the Medicines, Ethics and Practice Advisory Group. He completed his Clinical Diploma in Community Pharmacy at the University of Keele.

He can be found quite often on Twitter @Babir1981

Preface

Do you hate dilution calculations?

Then this is the book for you!

These 20 calculations with worked answers will ensure that your confidence with dilution calculations increases.

Always start at the end with dilutions and work backwards. The original concentration is always stronger or less dilute.

This book is not endorsed by the Royal Pharmaceutical Society or General Pharmaceutical Council.

Babir Malik

Acknowledgements

I would like to thank Joanna Domzal-Jamroz and Muniba Khalid for their kind assistance.

1. You need to prepare 300 mL of chlorhexidine gluconate 6 % w/v and have available a 50% w/v concentrate.

   How much concentrate, in mL, do you require?

						•			mL

2. What amount of copper sulphate, in mg, is required to make 400 mL of an aqueous stock solution, such that, when the stock solution is diluted 40 times with water, a final solution of 0.1% w/v copper sulphate is produced?

| | | | | | • | | | mg |

3. Potassium permanganate solution 1 in 8000 is prepared from a stock of 10 times this strength.

   How much potassium permanganate, in mg, will be needed to make sufficient stock solution if a patient uses 100 mL of the diluted solution each day for 3 days? Give your answer to one decimal place.

						•			mg

4. In your pharmacy you have a 100 mL bottle of stock solution of drug A with a concentration of 8% w/v. Drug A is used as a mouthwash at a concentration of 0.8% w/v twice daily. You are requested to supply 150 mL of a solution of intermediate strength, such that a 45-year-old patient will dilute this solution 1 in 5 to get the correct concentration immediately before use.

What is the concentration (% w/v) of the intermediate solution?

					•			% w/v

5. A patient needs to use a 1 in 400 chlorhexidine gluconate solution for wound washing. In your pharmacy you have a stock solution of 10% w/v chlorhexidine gluconate. Using this solution, you need to prepare an intermediate solution such that the patient will then dilute this 20-fold to obtain a solution of the requisite concentration.

What is the correct strength (% w/v) of the intermediate solution?

						•			% w/v

6. A patient needs to use a 1 in 2000 potassium permanganate solution for wound washing. In your pharmacy you have tablets of 400 mg potassium permanganate. Using (an) intact tablet(s) you need to prepare an intermediate solution such that the patient will then dilute this 20-fold to obtain a solution of the requisite concentration.

What is the correct strength of the intermediate solution in mg/mL?

						•			mg/mL

7. What mass of emulsifying ointment, in grams, needs to be added to 400 g of a 2 % w/w calamine in emulsifying ointment to produce a 0.1 % w/w calamine in emulsifying ointment?

						•			g

8. You receive the following request into your hospital manufacturing suite:

Send 500 mL benzalkonium chloride solution which when diluted 1 in 40 produces a 1 in 250 solution.

Assuming the only concentrated solution of benzalkonium chloride available contains 25% w/v, what volume of this concentrate is needed to fulfil the order?

					•			mL

9. When used as a foot soak, potassium permanganate is usually prepared as a stock solution, which is then diluted down. You are asked to prepare 50 mL of such stock solution, which, when 10 mL is diluted to 10 L, produces a final solution of 1 in 20,000.

How much potassium permanganate, in mg, is required?

						.			mg

10. How many micrograms of sodium fluoride are needed to prepare 200 mL of a sodium fluoride stock solution such that a solution containing 0.5 ppm of sodium fluoride results when 0.5 mL is diluted to 100 mL with water?

| | | | | | • | | | micrograms |

11. What weight of potassium permanganate, in grams, is required to produce 300 mL of a solution such that when 10 mL is diluted in 2 litres of water a 1 in 10,000 solution is produced?

						.			g

12. You have been asked to prepare 400 mL of a solution of miglustat concentrate, which when diluted with water 1 in 10, produces a 1 in 1,000 solution. You have in stock a 500 mL bottle of concentrate, which contains miglustat 20 %.

What volume of concentrate, mL, is required to complete the order?

					•			mL

13. You have been presented with a private prescription for 300 mL of a 0.02% w/v potassium permanganate cleansing solution. You check your stock and only have the 0.2% w/v potassium permanganate solution in stock.

    How many millilitres of 0.2% w/v potassium permanganate solution would be needed to make 300 millilitres of the more dilute solution, in order to fill the prescription?

						•			mL

14.   A stock solution of drug B is available at 50% w/v. You need to dilute this with Syrup BP to supply a patient with a solution containing 5 mg/mL of drug B.

Assuming no volume displacement effects, what quantity of syrup is needed, in mL, for the preparation of 100 mL of the final solution?

				•			mL

15. A stock solution of chlorhexidine acetate is available in 1 L bottles at a concentration of 0.07% w/v.

How many litres of purified water is required to be added to 20 mL of the stock solution to prepare a 5 ppm solution of chlorhexidine acetate for use as a wet dressing for the skin? Give your answer to TWO decimal places.

						•			L

16. The local chiropodist requires 400 mL of a potassium permanganate stock solution. When 10 mL of this stock solution is made up to 10 L with water, a final solution of 1 in 10,000 is required.

How much potassium permanganate powder, do you need to weigh out to make 400 mL of the stock solution?

					•			g

17.   If 50 g of a 2% w/w hydrocortisone ointment were diluted with 25 g of Vaseline, what would be the percentage concentration (% w/w) of hydrocortisone in the mixture? Give your answer to one decimal place

| | | | | | | . | | | % w/v |

18. A stock solution containing 10 mg/mL of drug A is used to prepare an intermediary solution such that when the intermediary solution is diluted 1 in 200, a 1 in 40,000 solution is obtained.

What volume of the stock solution, in mL, is required to supply 3 L of the intermediary solution?

					•			mL

19. You are required to prepare 300 mL of a solution of potassium permanganate of which when one part is diluted with seven parts of water makes a 1 in 4000 solution. This must be used as a foot soak.

How much potassium permanganate, in grams, is required? Give your answer to one decimal place.

						•			g

20.   You need to prepare 500 mL of an antiseptic solution such that when diluted 1 in 25 by the patient they will have a 0.01% solution to use. Your stock solution is 20%.

What volume of this in mL should be used? Give your answer to TWO decimal places.

					•			mL

1. You need to prepare 300 mL of chlorhexidine gluconate 6 % w/v and have available a 50% w/v concentrate.

How much concentrate, in mL, do you require?

				3	6	•			mL

Working 1

C1 x V1 = C2 x V2

C1 = 50 % w/v (the concentrate)

C2 = 6 % w/v (the concentration required after dilution)

V1 =? (volume of concentrate to use)

V2 = 300 mL (the volume required)

50 x V1 = 6 x 300

V1 = (6 x 300) ÷ 50

V1 = 1800 ÷ 50 = **36 mL**

Working 2

6% w/v = 6 g in 100 mL = 18 g in 300 mL

50% w/v = 50 g in 100 mL = 18 g in **36 mL**

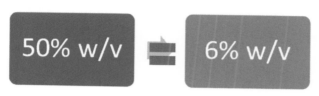

50% w/v
6% w/v

36 mL
Stock solution

300 mL
Final solution

2. What amount of copper sulphate, in mg, is required to make 400 mL of an aqueous stock solution, such that, when the stock solution is diluted 40 times with water, a final solution of 0.1% w/v copper sulphate is produced?

	1	6	0	0	0	•			mg

Working

If we work backwards from the final solution, we have 0.1% w/v, which equates to 0.1 g copper sulphate in 100 mL solution.

Multiplying by 40 gives the concentration of the original stock solution, which is, therefore, 4% w/v.

This equates to 4 g in 100 mL.

As we start with 400 mL stock solution, we need 4 g × 4, which is equal to 16 g copper sulphate

= 16,000 mg

Working 2

Initial concentration = final or weakest concentration × dilution factor

0.1% w/v x 40 = 4% w/v

4 g in 100 mL

16 g in 400 mL

16 g = 16,000 mg

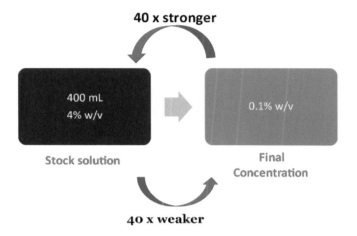

40 x stronger

400 mL
4% w/v

0.1% w/v

Stock solution

Final
Concentration

40 x weaker

3. Potassium permanganate solution 1 in 8000 is prepared from a stock of 10 times this strength.

   How much potassium permanganate, in mg, will be needed to make sufficient stock solution if a patient uses 100 mL of the diluted solution each day for 3 days? Give your answer to one decimal place.

			3	7	•	5		mg

Working 1

Of the diluted solution 300 mL will be used in 3 days.

If this solution has been prepared by a 10-fold dilution of the stock solution, the volume of the stock solution required must be 30 mL.

As the stock solution is a 1 in 800 solution, there would be 1 g or 1000 mg potassium permanganate in 800 mL.

In 30 mL there must be 0.0375 g or **37.5 mg** potassium permanganate

The question is asking for the amount and not the concentration.

Working 2

1 in 8000 = 1g in 8000 mL = 1000 mg in 8000 mL

1 mg in 8 mL = **37.5 mg** in 300 mL

Working 3

1 in 8000 = 0.0125% w/v

Stock is 10 times stronger so 1 in 800 = 0.125% w/v

C1 x V1 = C2 x V2

0.0125% w/v x 300 mL = 0.125% w/v x V2

V2 = 30 mL

So, 30 mL of 0.125% w/v

0.125 g in 100 mL

0.0375 g in 30 mL

37.5 mg in 30 mL

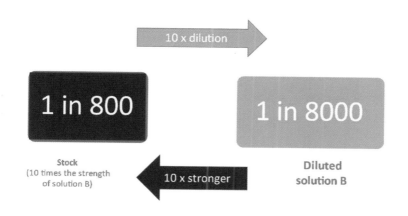

4. In your pharmacy you have a 100 mL bottle of stock solution of drug A with a concentration of 8% w/v. Drug A is used as a mouthwash at a concentration of 0.8% w/v twice daily. You are requested to supply 150 mL of a solution of intermediate strength, such that a 45-year-old patient will dilute this solution 1 in 5 to get the correct concentration immediately before use.

    What is the concentration (% w/v) of the intermediate solution?

				4	•			% w/v

Working 1

Drug A is used as a mouthwash at a concentration of 0.8% w/v.

If this has been prepared from a solution that has been diluted 1 in 5, multiplication by 5 gives the concentration of the intermediate solution, which is, therefore, **4% w/v.**

Working 2

Intermediate concentration = final concentration x dilution factor

0.08% w/v x 5 = **4% w/v**

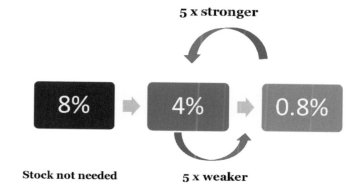

5. A patient needs to use a 1 in 400 chlorhexidine gluconate solution for wound washing. In your pharmacy you have a stock solution of 10% w/v chlorhexidine gluconate. Using this solution, you need to prepare an intermediate solution such that the patient will then dilute this 20-fold to obtain a solution of the requisite concentration.

What is the correct strength (% w/v) of the intermediate solution?

					5	•			% w/v

Working 1

Final solution = 1 in 100

Intermediate solution = (final concentration) × (dilution factor)

= (1 in 400) × (20) = 1 in 20

= 1 g in 20 mL

= 5 g in 100 mL

= **5% w/v**

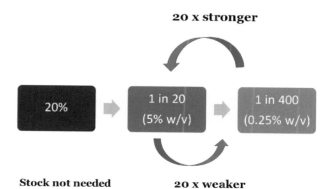

6. A patient needs to use a 1 in 2000 potassium permanganate solution for wound washing. In your pharmacy you have tablets of 400 mg potassium permanganate. Using (an) intact tablet(s) you need to prepare an intermediate solution such that the patient will then dilute this 20-fold to obtain a solution of the requisite concentration.

What is the correct strength of the intermediate solution in mg/mL?

				1	0	•			mg/mL

Working 1

The final solution for use by the patient = 1 in 2000

Intermediate solution = (final concentration) × (dilution factor)

= (1 in 2000) × (20) = 1 in 100

= 1 g in 100 mL

= 1000 mg in 100 mL

= 10 mg/mL

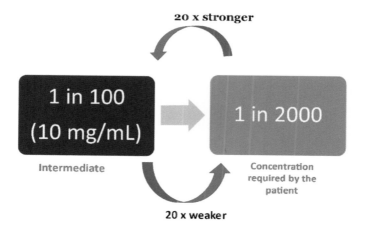

20 x stronger

1 in 100
(10 mg/mL)

Intermediate

1 in 2000

Concentration
required by the
patient

20 x weaker

7. What mass of emulsifying ointment, in grams, needs to be added to 400 g of a 2 % w/w calamine in emulsifying ointment to produce a 0.1 % w/w calamine in emulsifying ointment?

		7	6	0	0	•			g

Working

C1 x M1 = C2 x M2

C1 = 2% w/w

M1 = 400 g

C2 = 0.1% w/w

M2 =?

2 x 400 = 0.1 x M2

M2 = (2 x 400) ÷ 0.1

M2 = 800 ÷ 0.1

M2 = 8000 g

This means that 8000 g of 0.1 % w/w ointment contains the same amount of calamine as 400 g of 2 % w/w ointment.

Therefore, to make 8000 g of 0.1% w/w ointment you need to dilute 400 g of 2 % w/w with:

8000 – 400

= **7600 g** emulsifying ointment

8000 g − 400 g = 7600 g

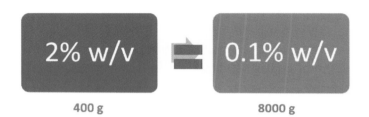

8. You receive the following request into your hospital manufacturing suite:

Send 500 mL benzalkonium chloride solution which when diluted 1 in 40 produces a 1 in 250 solution.

Assuming the only concentrated solution of benzalkonium chloride available contains 25% w/v, what volume of this concentrate is needed to fulfil the order?

			3	2	0	•			mL

Working 1

500 mL diluted 1 in 40 = 20,000 mL final solution

1 in 250 = 1 g in 250 mL = 80 g in 20,000 mL

20,000 mL will contain 80 g

Therefore, there is 80 g in the original 500 mL

The stock solution is 25 % w/v

= 25 g in 100 mL

= 1 g in 4 mL

= 80 g in **320 mL** stock needed.

Working 2

40-fold dilution so 1 in 250 (0.4%) ⮕ 1 in 6.25 (16%)

(500 mL x 16%) ÷ 25%

= 320 mL

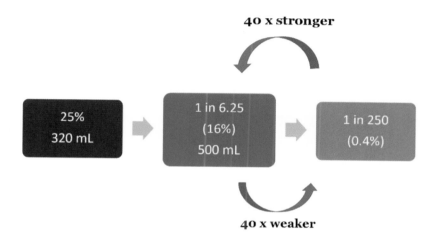

9. When used as a foot soak, potassium permanganate is usually prepared as a stock solution, which is then diluted down. You are asked to prepare 50 mL of such stock solution, which, when 10 mL is diluted to 10 L, produces a final solution of 1 in 20,000.

How much potassium permanganate, in mg, is required?

		2	5	0	0	•			mg

Working 1

10 mL —> 10,000 mL = 1000-fold dilution

1000 times stronger than 1 in 20,000 = 1 in 20

1 g in 20 mL

= 1000 mg in 20 mL

= **2500 mg** in 50 mL

Working 2

1 in 20000 = 1 g in 20000 mL

= 0.5 g in 10,000 mL

So, before dilution there was 0.5 g in 10 mL

0.5 g in 10 mL

2.5 g in 50 mL = **2500 mg** in 50 mL

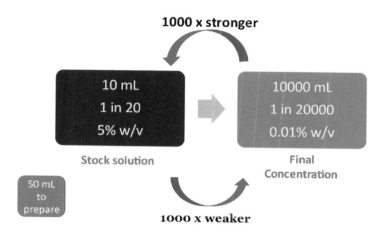

10. How many micrograms of sodium fluoride are needed to prepare 200 mL of a sodium fluoride stock solution such that a solution containing 0.5 ppm of sodium fluoride results when 0.5 mL is diluted to 100 mL with water?

	2	0	0	0	0	•			micrograms

Working 1

0.5 ppm = 0.5 g in 1,000,000 mL: Convert 0.5 g to micrograms

500,000 micrograms in 1,000,000 mL: Divide both sides by 10

50,000 micrograms in 100,000 mL: Divide both sides by 10

5,000 micrograms in 10,000 mL: Divide both sides by 10

500 micrograms in 1,000 mL: Divide both sides by 10

50 micrograms in 100 mL

Multiply 50 micrograms by 200 as this is the dilution factor (100 ÷ 0.5)

10,000 micrograms in 100 mL: Multiply both sides by 2

20,000 micrograms in 200 mL

Working 2

0.5 ppm = 0.5 g in 1,000,000 mL

= 0.00005 g in 100 mL

So, before dilution there was 0.00005 g in 0.5 mL

0.00005 g in 0.5 mL

0.02 g in 200 mL

20 mg in 200 mL

20,000 micrograms in 200 mL

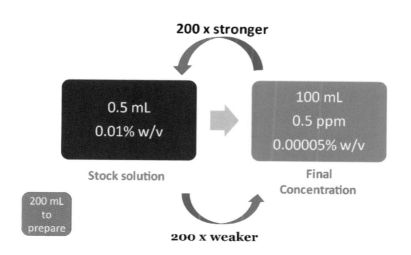

11. What weight of potassium permanganate, in grams, is required to produce 300 mL of a solution such that when 10 mL is diluted in 2 litres of water a 1 in 10,000 solution is produced?

					6	•			g

Working 1

10 mL to 2000 mL = 200-fold

1 in 10,000 x 200 = 1 in 50

6 g in 300 mL

Working 2

2000 mL ÷ 10 mL = 200 mL

1 in 10,000 = 0.01% w/v

0.01% w/v x 200 = 2% w/v

2 g in 100 mL

6 g in 300 mL

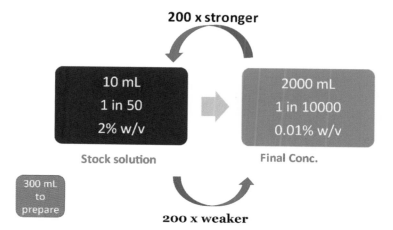

200 x stronger

10 mL	2000 mL
1 in 50	1 in 10000
2% w/v	0.01% w/v

Stock solution   Final Conc.

300 mL to prepare

200 x weaker

12. You have been asked to prepare 400 mL of a solution of miglustat concentrate, which when diluted with water 1 in 10, produces a 1 in 1,000 solution. You have in stock a 500 mL bottle of concentrate, which contains miglustat 20 %.

What volume of concentrate, mL, is required to complete the order?

				2	0	•			mL

Working 1

Diluted solution = 1 in 1,000, which has been diluted 10 times.

The concentrate is therefore 10 times stronger than this, i.e., 1 in 100

You need 400 mL of concentrate, therefore if 1 g in 100 mL, then 4 g in 400 mL

The miglustat is 20%, which is 20 g in 100 mL, or 1 g in 5 mL.

You need 4 g, which will be in **20 mL**

Working 2

1 in 1000 = 0.1% w/v

0.1% w/v x 10 (dilution factor) = 1% w/v

C1 x V1 = C2 x V2

$\dfrac{400 \text{ mL} \times 1}{20\% \text{ w/v}}$ = **20 mL**

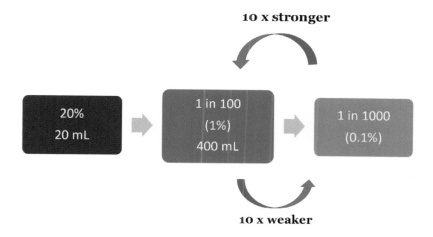

13. You have been presented with a private prescription for 300 mL of a 0.02% w/v potassium permanganate cleansing solution. You check your stock and only have the 0.2% w/v potassium permanganate solution in stock.

How many millilitres of 0.2% w/v potassium permanganate solution would be needed to make 300 millilitres of the more dilute solution, in order to fill the prescription?

			3	0	•			mL

Working 1

C1 x V1 = C2 x V2

0.2% x V1 = 0.02% x 300 mL

V1 = (0.02% x 300 mL) ÷ 0.2%

= 30 mL

Working 2

0.02% w/v = 0.06 g in 300 mL

0.2% w/v = 0.06 g in **30 mL**

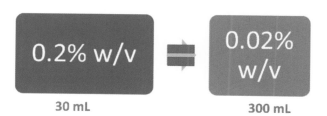

0.2% w/v ⇒ 0.02% w/v

30 mL · 300 mL

14.	A stock solution of drug B is available at 50% w/v. You need to dilute this with Syrup BP to supply a patient with a solution containing 5 mg/mL of drug B.

Assuming no volume displacement effects, what quantity of syrup is needed, in mL, for the preparation of 100 mL of the final solution?

			9	9	•			mL

Working 1

The stock solution = 50% w/v = 50 g in 100 mL

= 50,000 mg in 100 mL = 500 mg/mL.

The solution supplied to the patient is 5 mg/mL and so a 1 in 100 dilution must be performed.

1 mL of the stock solution should be diluted to 100 mL with **99 mL Syrup BP.**

Working 2

5 mg/mL = 500 mg/100 mL = 0.5%

0.5% x 100 divided 50 = 1 mL

So 1 mL of 5mg/mL and **99 mL syrup**

100 mL – 1 mL = 99 mL

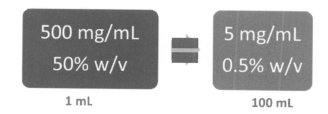

500 mg/mL
50% w/v

5 mg/mL
0.5% w/v

1 mL   100 mL

15.   A stock solution of chlorhexidine acetate is available in 1 L bottles at a concentration of 0.07% w/v.

How many litres of purified water is required to be added to 20 mL of the stock solution to prepare a 5 ppm solution of chlorhexidine acetate for use as a wet dressing for the skin? Give your answer to TWO decimal places.

				2	•	7	8	L

Working 1

0.07 % = 0.07 g in 100 mL = 0.014 g in 20 mL

5 ppm = 5 g in 1,000,000 mL

$\qquad$ = 1 g in 200,000 mL

$\qquad$ = 0.001 g in 20 mL

$\qquad$ = 0.014 g in 2800 mL

Therefore 2800 mL – 20 mL = 2780 mL = **2.78 L**

Working 2

50 ppm = 5 g in 1,000,000 mL

= 0.5 g in 100,000 mL

= 0.05 g in 10,000 mL

= 0.005 g in 1,000 mL

= 0.0005 g in 100 mL

(20 mL x 0.07%) ÷ 0.0005%

= 2800 mL

2800 mL – 20 mL = 2780 mL = **2.78 L**

2800 mL - 20 mL = 2780 mL = 2.78 L

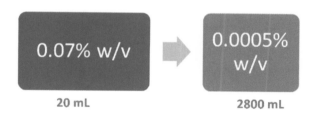

0.07% w/v → 0.0005% w/v

20 mL   2800 mL

16.   The local chiropodist requires 400 mL of a potassium permanganate stock solution.   When 10 mL of this stock solution is made up to 10 L with water, a final solution of 1 in 10,000 is required.

How much potassium permanganate powder, do you need to weigh out to make 400 mL of the stock solution?

			4	0	•			g

Working 1

10 mL in 10 L = 10 mL in 10,000 mL = 1 in 1000

Final Solution is 1 in 10,000 which is a 1 in 10 dilution of the 1 in 1000 stock solution

1 in 10 = 1 g in 10 mL = 10 g in 100 mL

= **40 g** in 400 mL

Working 2

$C_1V_1 = C_2V_2$

C_1x 10 mL = 1 in 10000 x 10 L

C_1 x 10 mL = 0.01% x 10,000 mL

C_1 = 0.01% x 10,000 mL ÷ 10 mL = 10% w/v

400 mL of 10% solution contains 10 g in 100 mL

= **40 g** in 400 mL

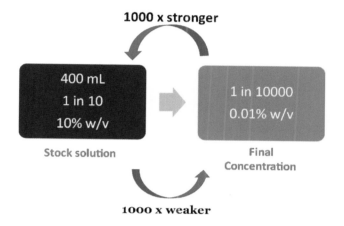

17.   If 50 g of a 2% w/w hydrocortisone ointment were diluted with 25 g of Vaseline, what would be the percentage concentration (% w/w) of hydrocortisone in the mixture? Give your answer to one decimal place.

				1	•	3		% w/v

Working 1

50 g + 25 g = 75 g

C1V1

50 g x 2% = C2 x 75 g

50 x 2 ÷ 75 g = **1.3% w/w** to one decimal place

Working 2

2% = 2 g in 100 g so 1 g in 50 g

This was added to 25 g Vaseline so 1 g in 75 g

1 g in 75 g = 1.3 g in 100 g = **1.3% w/w**

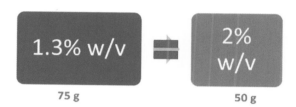

1.3% w/v = 2% w/v

75 g   50 g

18.   A stock solution containing 10 mg/mL of drug A is used to prepare an intermediary solution such that when the intermediary solution is diluted 1 in 200, a 1 in 40,000 solution is obtained.

What volume of the stock solution, in mL, is required to supply 3 L of the intermediary solution?

	1	5	0	0	•			mL

Working

Intermediate solution is 200 times stronger than the final concentration 1 in 40,000

So 1 in 200

1 in 200 = 1 g in 200 mL

So 0.5 g in 100 mL so 0.5%

Stock solution is 10 mg/mL so 1,000 mg in 100 mL so 1%

C1V1 = 1% x V1 = 0.5% x 3000 mL

V1 = **1500 mL**

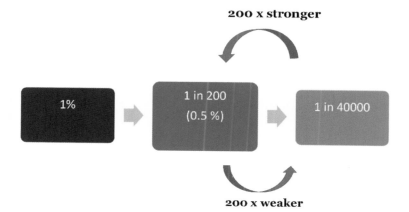

19.   You are required to prepare 300 mL of a solution of potassium permanganate of which when one part is diluted with seven parts of water makes a 1 in 4000 solution. This must be used as a foot soak.

How much potassium permanganate, in grams, is required? Give your answer to one decimal place.

					0	•	6		g

Working

Final strength is 1 in 4000

To get here 'Original strength' has been diluted one part (1) with (+) 7 parts water therefore it is 8 times weaker

Therefore 'original strength' is 4000 divided by 8 = 1 in 500

Quantity potassium permanganate: 1 g in 500 mL

                                        0.2 g in 100 mL

            Therefore   **0.6 g** in 300 mL

Working 2

1 in 4000 = 0.025% w/v

0.025% w/v x 8 = 0.2% w/v

0.2 g in 100 mL so **0.6 g** in 300 mL

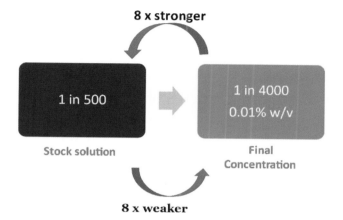

8 x stronger

1 in 500

Stock solution

1 in 4000
0.01% w/v

Final
Concentration

8 x weaker

20. You need to prepare 500 mL of an antiseptic solution such that when diluted 1 in 25 by the patient they will have a 0.01% solution to use. Your stock solution is 20%.

What volume of this in mL should be used? Give your answer to TWO decimal places.

					6	•	2	5	mL

Working 1

The solution will be 0.01% when diluted 1 in 25

Therefore, the solution before dilution will be 0.01 x 25 = 0.25%

20% x V1 = 0.25% x 500 mL

20% x V1 = 125

V1 = 125 ÷ 20 = **6.25 mL**

Working 2

0.25% w/v = 0.25 g in 100 mL = 1.25 g in 500 mL

20% w/v = 20 g in 100 mL = 1.25 g in **6.25 mL**

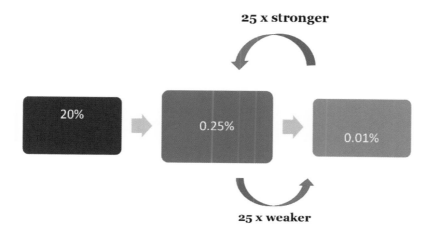

Printed in Great Britain
by Amazon